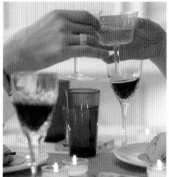

food for
Lovers

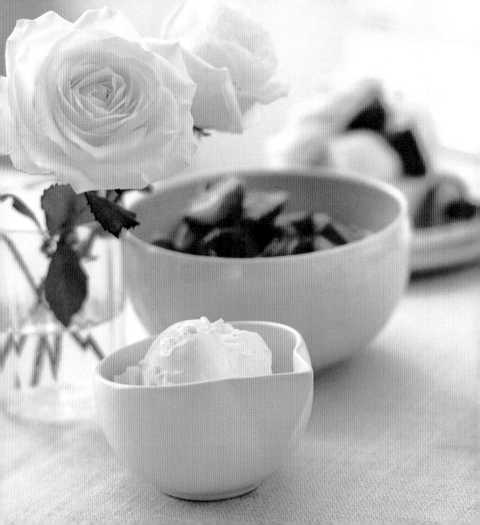

food for
Lovers

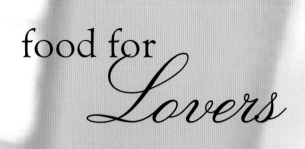

RYLAND
PETERS
& SMALL

LONDON NEW YORK

Designer Sarah Fraser

Commissioning Editor
Elsa Petersen-Schepelern

Editor Sharon Cochrane

Picture Research Emily Westlake

Production Sheila Smith and
Deborah Wehner

Art Director Gabriella Le Grazie

Publishing Director Alison Starling

Index Hilary Bird

Notes

All spoon measurements are level unless
otherwise specified.

All eggs are medium unless otherwise
specified. Uncooked or partly cooked
eggs should not be served to the
very young, the very old, those with
compromised immune systems or
to pregnant women.

Ovens should be preheated to the specified
temperature. If using a fan-assisted oven,
cooking times should be reduced according
to the manufacturer's instructions.

First published in the
United Kingdom in 2006
by Ryland Peters & Small
20–21 Jockey's Fields
London WC1R 4BW
www.rylandpeters.com

10 9 8 7 6 5 4 3 2 1

ISBN-13: 978 1 84172 961 9
ISBN-10: 1 84172 961 2

A CIP catalogue record for this book is
available from the British Library.

Printed in China

Contents

Aphrodisiac Foods

For centuries many cultures have believed that certain foods possess aphrodisiac qualities – from the Aztecs who thought their highly prized chocolate enhanced sexual prowess, to the Romans who considered garlic capable of stimulating sexual desire.

Whether it's chocolate or oysters, asparagus or strawberries, aphrodisiac foods are a sure-fire way to revive any relationship. The recipes in this book are designed to set your desire alight, so if you think your relationship needs a boost, get cooking and bring the flames of passion to life.

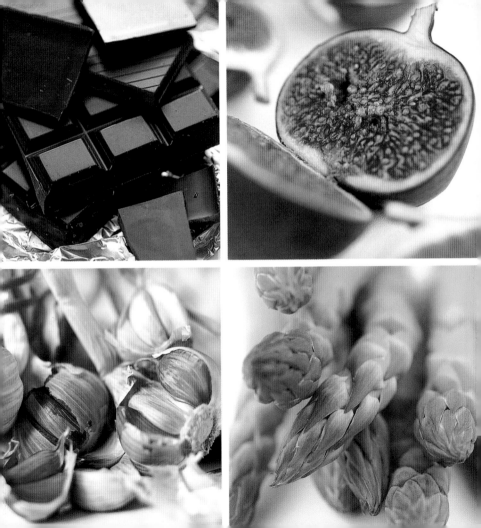

Apricots *are a blushing fruit, considered a symbol of sensuality by the ancient Chinese*

Asparagus *is regarded by several cultures as a stimulant because of its erotic shape*

Bananas *have a suggestive shape, but also contain sex hormone-producing minerals*

Champagne *there's something in the bubbles*

Cherries *are very sensual, especially when dipped in melted chocolate*

Chocolate *legend says that the Aztec Emperor Montezuma drank 50 cups of frothy xocolatl before visiting his harem*

Eggs, *including caviar, stimulate the libido*

Figs *are erotic, fleshy fruits said to act as a powerful sexual stimulant*

Garlic *was considered an aphrodisiac by the Greeks, Egyptians, Romans, Chinese and Japanese*

Ginger *stimulates the circulatory system and gets you 'in the mood'*

Honey *is a derivation of the word 'honeymoon', during which the couple would drink mead (honey wine)*

Liquorice *is said to enhance love and lust, especially in women*

Nuts, *particularly pine nuts, have been used for centuries to make up love potions*

Oysters *Casanova was said to eat 50 of them each morning to enhance his sexual prowess*

Peaches *make a sensuous treat with their curvaceous shape and succulent texture*

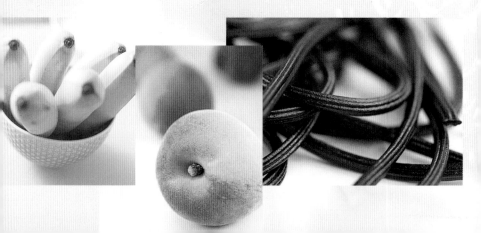

Red meat *will give you the strength you need for a night of passion*

Rose petals *are the epitome of edible romance*

Saffron *is widely used as an aphrodisiac in Asia and the Middle East*

Seafood *is high in phosphorus, iodine and often zinc, which increase sexual potency*

Strawberries *are regarded as a powerful stimulant – the perfect finger food for lovers*

Tomatoes *are known as the 'love apple' in French – say no more…*

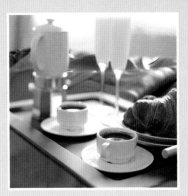

Breakfast in Bed

The way to a man's heart is through his stomach.
Fanny Fern (1811–1872)

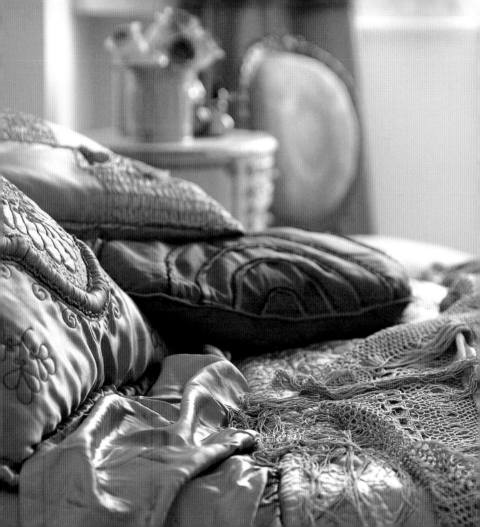

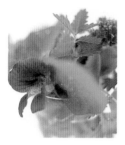

Stirring a little creamy goats' cheese into lightly scrambled eggs transforms a simple dish into something special enough to serve for breakfast in bed. The nasturtium flowers add a touch of romance as well as a delightful flash of colour.

creamy eggs
with goats' cheese

6 free-range eggs

50 ml single cream

1 tablespoon chopped fresh marjoram

25 g butter

100 g goats' cheese, diced

a small handful of nasturtium flowers, torn (optional)

sea salt and freshly ground black pepper

toasted walnut bread, to serve

serves 2

Put the eggs, cream, marjoram and a little salt and pepper in a bowl and beat well. Melt the butter in a non-stick saucepan, add the eggs and stir over low heat until the eggs begin to set.

Stir in the goats' cheese and continue to cook briefly, stirring all the time, until the cheese melts into the eggs. Add the nasturtium flowers, if using, and spoon onto the toast. Serve immediately.

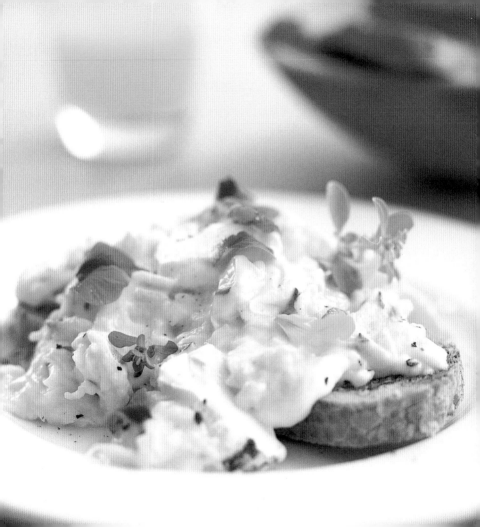

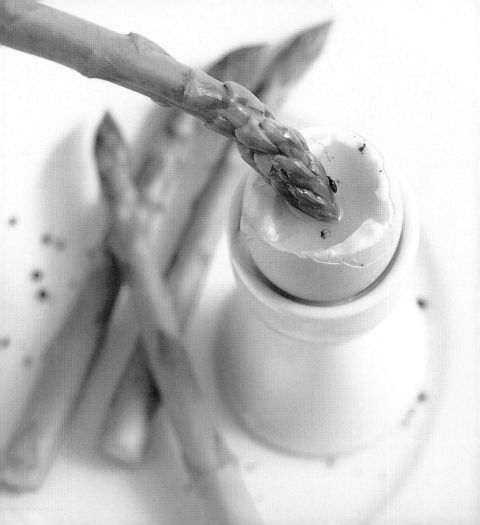

Dunking toast into the perfect soft-boiled egg is one of the simple pleasures in life. Well, it's even better when you dip in asparagus spears – and it's much more sensual, too.

soft cooked eggs
with asparagus soldiers

Tie the asparagus into 2 bunches of 6 with string. Steam or boil it for 3–4 minutes until just tender. Drain and keep warm.

Meanwhile, cook the eggs in gently boiling water for 4 minutes, then transfer them to egg cups. Remove the tops of the eggs with a knife and sprinkle with salt and pepper to taste. Serve with the asparagus and some toast, if liked.

12 thick asparagus spears

4 large free-range eggs, at room temperature

sea salt and freshly ground black pepper

toast, to serve (optional)

egg cups

serves 2

honey-roasted peaches
with ricotta and coffee bean sugar

This is a mouthwatering recipe, to be enjoyed on a warm summer morning. Grinding whole coffee beans with lump sugar is typically Italian and adds a delicious crunch to the dish.

Put the peach or nectarine halves, cut side up, in the prepared baking dish. Drizzle with the honey and roast in a preheated oven at 220°C (425°F) Gas 7 for 15–20 minutes, until the fruit is tender and caramelized. Remove from the oven and let cool slightly.

Put the coffee beans and sugar in a coffee grinder and blitz very briefly, until the beans and sugar are coarsely ground.

Spoon the peaches or nectarines onto plates, top with a scoop of ricotta and a sprinkle of the sugary coffee beans, then serve.

2 large peaches or nectarines, halved and stones removed

1 tablespoon clear honey

1 teaspoon coffee beans

1 teaspoon rough sugar pieces or 2 sugar lumps

100 g ricotta cheese, chilled

a baking dish lined with baking parchment

serves 2

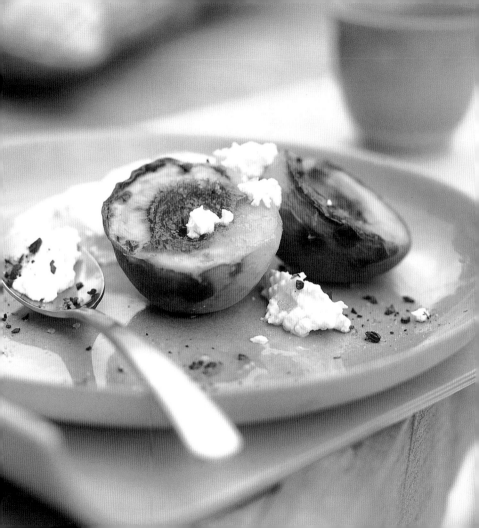

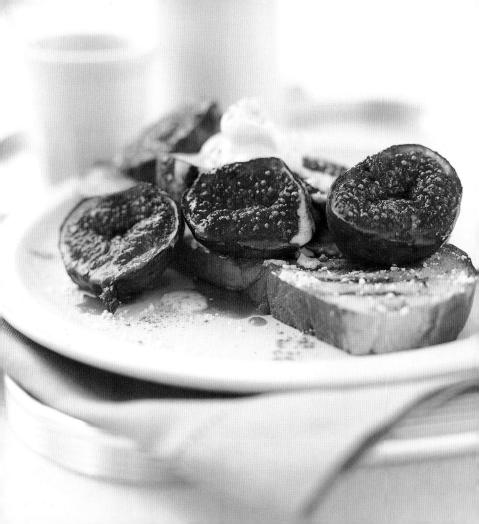

sweet bruschetta *with figs*

1 tablespoon
quince paste*

15 g butter

1 tablespoon port

6 ripe figs, halved

2 slices of brioche loaf
or challah

icing sugar, for dusting

cinnamon, for dusting

Greek yoghurt, to serve

serves 2

Juicy fresh figs are a sweet – and sensual – breakfast treat. The quince is also considered to be a food for lovers.

Put the quince paste, butter and port in a small saucepan and heat gently until melted. Put the figs, cut side up, in an ovenproof dish. Spoon over the port mixture, making sure the surface of each fig is well covered. Put the figs under a preheated hot grill and cook for 3–5 minutes, until they are caramelized and heated through.

Meanwhile, toast the brioche or challah on a stove-top grill pan. Transfer to heated serving plates and sprinkle immediately with icing sugar and cinnamon. Top with the figs and serve with a spoonful of Greek yoghurt.

*Note Quince paste is available from specialist food stores. If you can't find it, use redcurrant jelly or raspberry jam instead.

red berry sauce

3 punnets strawberries, about 700 g

1 tablespoon freshly squeezed lemon juice

4 tablespoons sugar

waffle batter

250 g plain flour

1/4 teaspoon salt

1/2 tablespoon baking powder

2 eggs, separated

1 tablespoon butter, melted

250 ml milk

to serve

500 ml strawberry ice cream

icing sugar, for dusting

an electric 4-heart-patterned waffle iron, greased

a heart-shaped biscuit cutter

serves 4

These heart-shaped waffles make a deliciously romantic start to the day.

waffle hearts

To make the red berry sauce, put the strawberries, lemon juice and sugar in a saucepan and heat gently until the juices run. When the berries have become pale and the juice dark, push them through a plastic sieve or simply strain the juice. Set aside.

To make the waffle batter, sift the flour, salt and baking powder into a bowl and make a well in the centre. Beat the egg yolks until creamy. Beat the egg whites in a second bowl until stiff and frothy. Pour the melted butter into the flour, then the egg yolks and milk. Mix well, then fold in the beaten egg whites.

Heat the waffle iron until faintly smoking. Pour a little batter into each compartment and spread over quickly. Close the waffle iron and leave for 1 minute until golden brown. Transfer the waffle to a heated plate and cook the remaining mixture in the same way. Break the waffles into the heart segments.

Using the biscuit cutter, make 4 strawberry ice cream hearts 4 cm thick. Put a waffle heart on a chilled plate, top with an ice cream heart, then a second waffle heart. Drizzle with about 1 tablespoon red berry sauce, dust with icing sugar and serve.

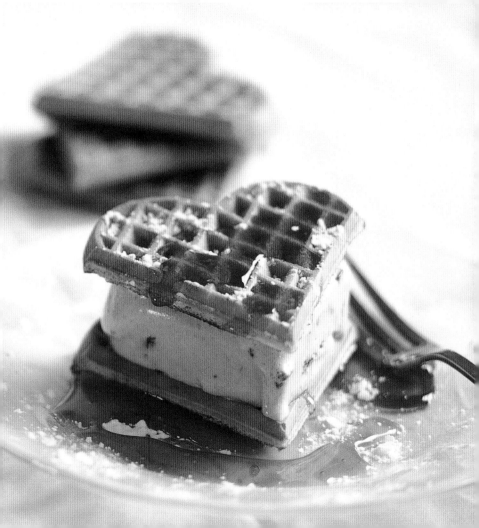

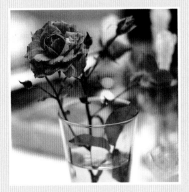

Romantic Dinners

Whosoever says truffle, utters a grand word, which awakens erotic and gastronomic ideas...
Jean-Anthelme Brillat-Savarin (1755–1826)

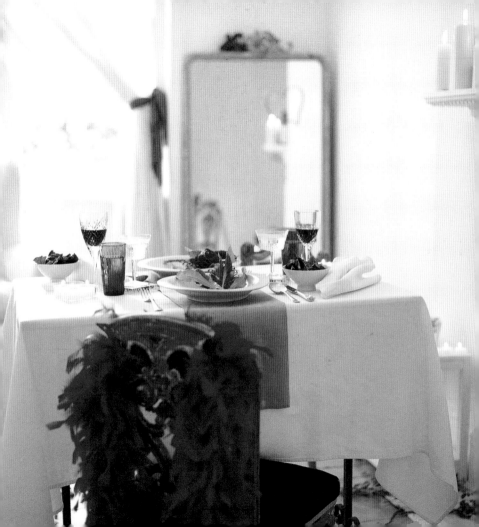

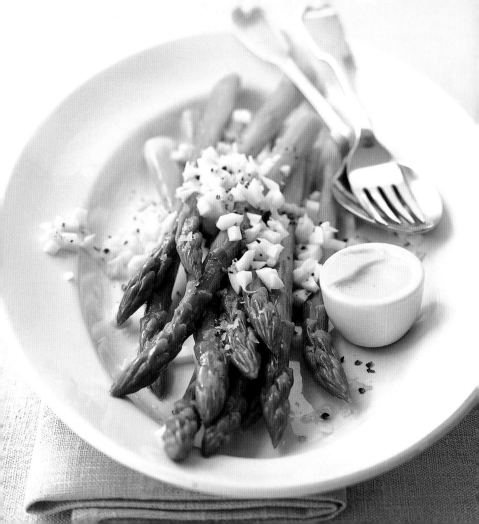

The truffle oil is an optional luxury but it is wonderful with egg and asparagus, and it will help boost the passion levels, too. Truffles were much prized by the Romans for their erotic powers, so do use the oil if you can.

asparagus *with egg and truffle butter*

2 free-range eggs

50 g unsalted butter, softened

a little truffle oil (optional)

250 g fresh asparagus, trimmed

sea salt and freshly ground black pepper

serves 2

Hard-boil the eggs for about 10 minutes, depending on their size. Let cool in cold water, then peel them. Halve the eggs and remove the yolks. Finely chop the whites and reserve. Mash the yolks with the butter until well blended. Add a drop or two of truffle oil, if using, and season with salt. Cover and keep at room temperature.

Steam the asparagus for about 12 minutes until tender. Arrange on 2 warm plates, sprinkle with the chopped egg white and salt and pepper, then serve with the golden butter. (The butter can be either spooned on top to melt into the spears or served in little dishes to spread onto each mouthful.)

Oysters are the ultimate aphrodisiac. Purists would never serve their oysters any way but naked (the oysters, that is), but the Thai dressing adds some spice.

fresh oysters *with thai dressing*

To make the dressing, put the lemongrass, lime leaf, fish sauce, lime juice, mirin and sugar in a blender, then add 1 tablespoon water. Blend well, then set aside to infuse for 2 hours. Strain into a clean bowl and stir in the cucumber and coriander.

To shuck the oysters, put them cupped side down on a flat work surface. Insert a knife into the hinge and twist it until the top shell is loosened, then twist it off, reserving as much of the juice as possible. Spoon the dressing over the oysters and serve at once on a bed of ice.

12 fresh oysters

ice cubes, to serve

thai dressing

1 stalk of lemongrass, very thinly sliced

1 kaffir lime leaf, very thinly sliced, or the finely grated zest of $^1/_2$ unwaxed lime

1 tablespoon Thai fish sauce

$^3/_4$ tablespoon freshly squeezed lime juice

$^3/_4$ tablespoon mirin (sweetened Japanese rice wine)

$^1/_2$ teaspoon caster sugar

3 cm piece of cucumber, peeled and diced

a few coriander leaves

serves 2

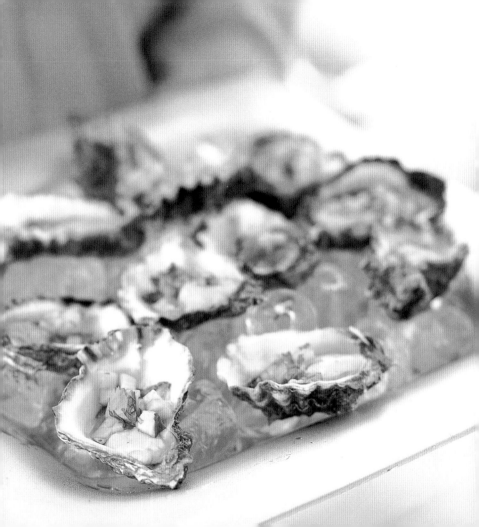

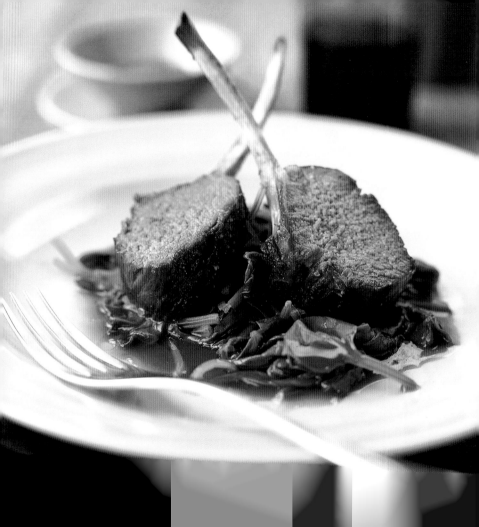

rack of lamb

1 rack of lamb

about 250 g baby spinach, wilted

marinating syrup

1 tablespoon redcurrant jelly

75 ml sweet sherry

75 ml sherry vinegar

1 $^1/_2$ tablespoons sugar

1 tablespoon soy sauce

1 sprig of rosemary

1 small garlic clove, sliced

gravy

15 g unsalted butter

75 ml white vermouth

125 ml lamb or chicken stock

sea salt and freshly ground black pepper

non-stick baking parchment or kitchen foil

a roasting tin

serves 2

To make the marinating syrup, put the redcurrant jelly in a saucepan, add the sherry, vinegar, sugar, soy sauce, rosemary and 2 slices of the garlic and boil to reduce and form a syrup. Brush the syrup all over the rack of lamb and put it in a plastic bag with the rest of the syrup. Set aside to marinate for 2 hours, turning every 30 minutes.

When ready to cook, wipe the excess marinade off the rack of lamb, reserving the marinade. Set the lamb on non-stick baking parchment or a sheet of kitchen foil in a roasting tin and roast in a preheated oven at 250°C (500°F) Gas 9 for 8 minutes. Remove from the oven and let rest in a warm place for up to 2 hours.

To serve, reheat the rack for 6–8 minutes in the very hot oven, then slice it between the bones. Put a bed of cooked spinach on each plate, then put the cutlets on top, crossing over the bones.

Meanwhile, to make the gravy, put the butter in a small saucepan, add the vermouth and boil until reduced by half. Add the stock and 1–2 teaspoons of the leftover marinade, bring to the boil and reduce again to improve the flavour. Season to taste with salt and pepper, pour around the meat, then serve immediately.

steak and chips

250 g floury potatoes (for baking and frying), peeled and cut into 5 mm slices

sunflower oil for deep-frying, plus 1/2 tablespoon

2 sirloin or rib eye steaks, about 300 g each, 3 cm thick

sea salt and freshly ground black pepper

shallot butter

50 g unsalted butter, softened

1 shallot, finely chopped

75 ml red wine

a large sprig of tarragon

several sprigs of flat leaf parsley

1/2 teaspoon sea salt

1/4 teaspoon coarsely ground black pepper

a large saucepan with frying basket, or an electric deep-fryer

serves 2

To make the shallot butter, melt half of the butter very gently in a saucepan. Add the shallot and cook until softened. Add the wine, bring to the boil and cook until syrupy and the wine has almost completely evaporated. Let cool. Put the cooled shallot, remaining butter, tarragon, parsley, salt and pepper in a small food processor and blend briefly. Transfer to a piece of baking parchment and roll up into a log shape. Chill until firm.

To make the chips, cut the potato slices into 5 mm strips. Put in a bowl of iced water for at least 5 minutes. Drain and pat dry. Fill a large saucepan one-third full with oil, or if using a deep-fryer to the manufacturer's recommended level. Heat the oil to 190°C (375°F) or until a cube of bread browns in 30 seconds. Working in batches, put 2 handfuls of potato strips in the frying basket, lower into the oil and fry for about 4 minutes. Remove and drain on kitchen paper. Repeat with the remaining strips. Reheat the oil to 190°C (375°F), then fry the strips for a second time until crisp and golden, about 2 minutes. Drain on kitchen paper, sprinkle with salt and keep warm.

Rub the steaks on both sides with the oil. Heat a ridged stove-top grill pan, add the steaks and cook for 1 1/2–2 minutes on each side for a rare steak, or for 3 1/2–4 minutes on each side for medium-rare. Remove from the pan and season both sides. Let stand for a few minutes, then serve with the butter and chips.

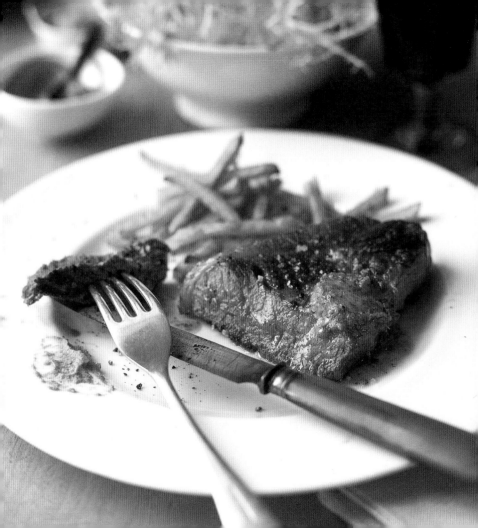

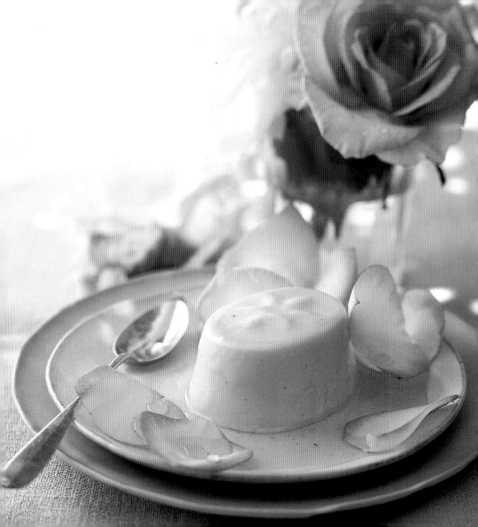

panna cotta *with rose petal syrup*

1 sachet gelatine granules,
about 7 g

150 ml single cream

1 vanilla pod, split
lengthways, seeds removed
with the point of a knife

75 g caster sugar

500 g mascarpone cheese

$\frac{1}{2}$ teaspoon almond
extract or 1 tablespoon
Amaretto liqueur

1 teaspoon rosewater

syrup

25 g vanilla sugar

6–8 tablespoons white wine

to serve

petals of 1 scented rose

6–8 cantucci or amaretti
biscuits (optional)

6–8 small pots, cups
or dishes, 100–125 ml
each, oiled

serves 6–8

Put the gelatine in a heatproof bowl, add 4 tablespoons water and leave to swell.

Put the cream, vanilla pod and its seeds in a small saucepan, heat to simmering, then almost to boiling, then turn off the heat. Let stand for 2 minutes. Stir in the soaked gelatine until it dissolves. Remove the vanilla pod (you can dry it and use it to perfume a jar of sugar, if liked).

Put the sugar, mascarpone, almond extract or Amaretto liqueur and $\frac{1}{2}$ teaspoon of the rosewater in a bowl and whisk until creamy and smooth. Whisk in the gelatine mixture. Pour into the prepared pots, cups or dishes and chill for at least 2 hours.

Meanwhile, to make the syrup, put the vanilla sugar and white wine in a small saucepan, heat over low heat and stir until dissolved and bubbling. Let cool slightly, then stir in the remaining rosewater.

Serve the panna cotta in their pots, or turned out, with a trickle of syrup and several scented rose petals, and crisp biscuits such as cantucci or amaretti.

rose petal tart

350 g frozen puff pastry, thawed

150 g Greek yoghurt

1 egg yolk

2–3 tablespoons rosewater

2 tablespoons caster sugar

300 ml double cream, whisked until soft peaks form

crystallized rose petals

1 egg white

petals of 2–4 scented roses

caster sugar

a wire rack or non-stick baking parchment

a round or heart-shaped tart tin, 25 cm diameter

foil and baking beans

makes a 25 cm tart

To crystallize the rose petals, put the egg white in a bowl, beat until frothy, then paint onto clean dry petals. Sprinkle with caster sugar to coat completely, then arrange on a wire rack or non-stick baking parchment and leave in a warm place to dry out and crisp – at least overnight. Let cool, but do not put in the refrigerator. Store between layers of kitchen paper in an airtight container.

Roll out the pastry as thinly as possible and line the tart tin with it, trimming to leave 5 mm hanging over the edge. Turn this inwards to make a rim. Prick the base all over with a fork, then chill or freeze for 15 minutes. Line with foil and baking beans and bake blind in a preheated oven at 230°C (450°F) Gas 8 for 12–15 minutes. Remove the foil and beans and reduce the temperature to 200°C (400°F) Gas 6. Return the pastry case to the oven for 5 minutes more to dry out. You may have to flatten the pastry if it puffs up.

Reduce the temperature to 180°C (350°F) Gas 4. Put the yoghurt, egg yolk, rosewater and sugar in a bowl and mix. Fold in the whisked cream. Spoon into the pastry case, level the surface and bake for 20 minutes. It will seem almost runny, but will set as it cools. Cover and chill until firm. Decorate with the crystallized rose petals. Serve slightly cold.

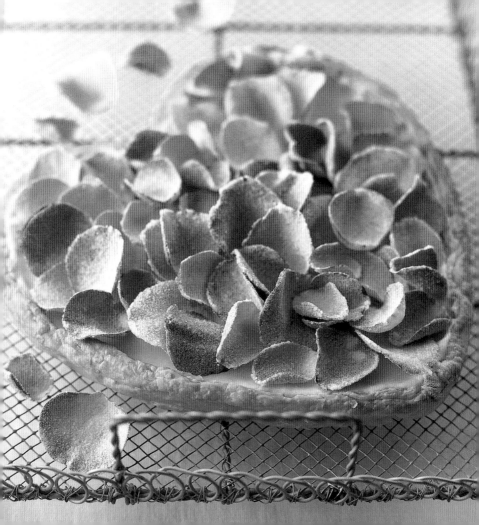

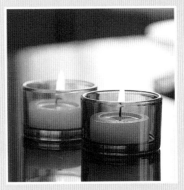

Cosy Suppers

*Men become passionately attached to women who
know how to cosset them with delicate tidbits.*
Honoré de Balzac (1799–1859)

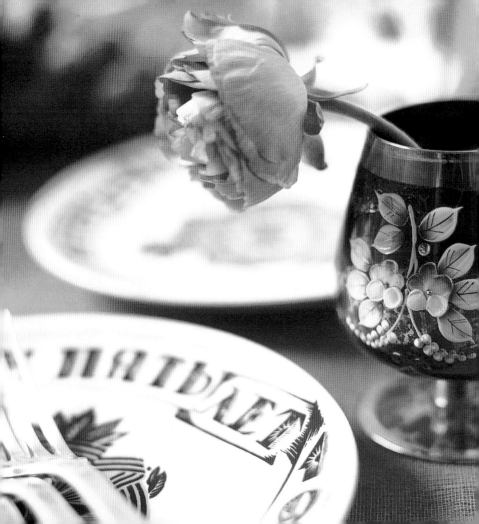

This is a hands-on dish that's perfect for an intimate supper for two. Serve these prawns with lots of fresh, crusty bread to mop up the garlicky sauce.

garlic prawns

75 ml olive oil

500 g prawn tails, with shells

4-5 garlic cloves, chopped

a handful of flat leaf parsley, chopped

sea salt and freshly ground black pepper

1 lemon, cut into wedges, to serve

serves 2

Heat the oil in a large sauté pan. When hot but not smoking, add the prawns and garlic and cook for 3-5 minutes until the prawns turn pink. Be careful not to let the garlic burn. Remove the pan from the heat, sprinkle the prawns with salt, pepper and parsley and mix well. Serve immediately, with lemon wedges.

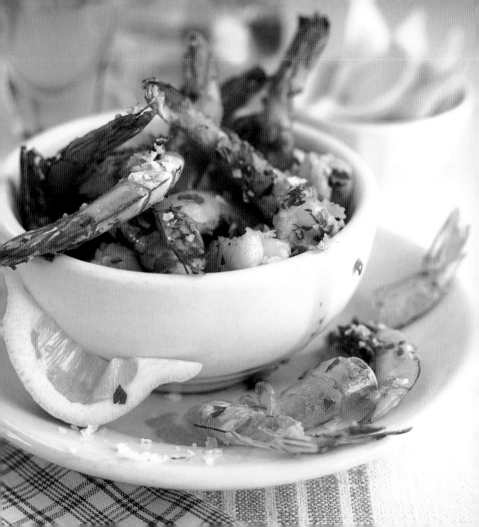

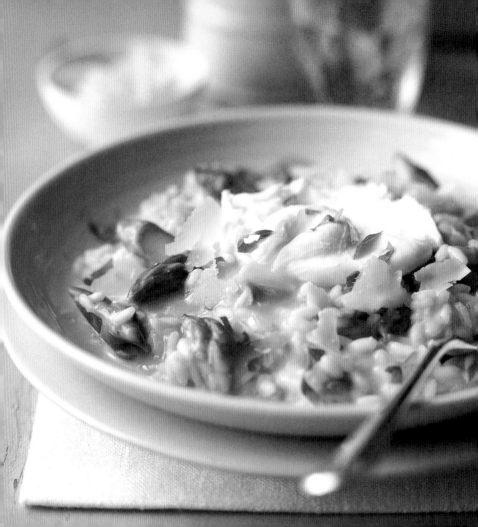

asparagus risotto

Put the hot stock in a wide saucepan. Add the asparagus and boil for about 6 minutes until tender. Drain, reserving the stock and transferring it to a regular saucepan to simmer. Plunge the asparagus into cold water, then drain and cut it into small pieces.

To poach the eggs, fill a saucepan with boiling water. Add the vinegar, then give it a stir to create a whirlpool. Slip an egg into the vortex, then simmer for 2–3 minutes. Using a slotted spoon, transfer the poached egg to a pan of warm water. Repeat with the other eggs. Keep them warm while you make the risotto.

Melt half the butter in a large, heavy saucepan and add the shallots. Cook gently for 5–6 minutes until soft and translucent but not browned. Add the rice and stir until well coated with the butter and heated through. Begin adding the hot stock, a large ladle at a time, stirring gently until each ladle has almost been absorbed by the rice. The risotto should be kept at a bare simmer throughout, so don't let the rice dry out – add more stock as necessary. Continue until the rice is tender and creamy, but the grains still firm, 15–20 minutes.

Beat in the Parmesan, the remaining butter and salt and pepper, to taste. Fold in the drained asparagus. Cover, let rest for a few minutes, then serve topped with a drained poached egg, some parsley and tarragon and Parmesan shavings.

about 1.5 litres hot vegetable or chicken stock

500 g fresh green or purple-tipped asparagus, trimmed

1 teaspoon tarragon or white wine vinegar

6 free-range eggs, cracked into separate cups

125 g unsalted butter

2 large shallots, finely chopped

500 g risotto rice, preferably carnaroli

50 g freshly grated Parmesan cheese

sea salt and freshly ground black pepper

to serve

1 tablespoon chopped fresh parsley and tarragon, mixed

Parmesan cheese shavings

serves 6

This is easy to make and ideal for a cosy supper, since it should be made one day in advance. You should use good-quality chocolate, but anything over 70 per cent cocoa solids will be too much.

chocolate mousse

200 g plain chocolate (70 per cent cocoa solids), broken into pieces

30 g unsalted butter, cut into small pieces

1 vanilla pod, split lengthways

3 eggs, separated

a pinch of salt

2 tablespoons caster sugar

sweetened crème fraîche or whipped cream, to serve (optional)

serves 4

Put the chocolate in a heatproof glass bowl and melt in the microwave on High for 40 seconds. Remove, stir and repeat until almost completely melted. Remove, then stir in the butter. Using the tip of a small sharp knife, scrape the seeds from the vanilla pod into the chocolate. Add the egg yolks, stir and set aside.

Put the egg whites and salt in a large, grease-free bowl and, using an electric mixer, beat until foaming. Continue beating and add the sugar. Beat on high until the mixture is glossy and firm.

Carefully fold the whites into the chocolate with a rubber spatula until no more white specks can be seen.

Transfer the mousse to serving dishes and refrigerate for at least 6 hours, preferably overnight. Serve with sweetened crème fraîche or whipped cream, if liked.

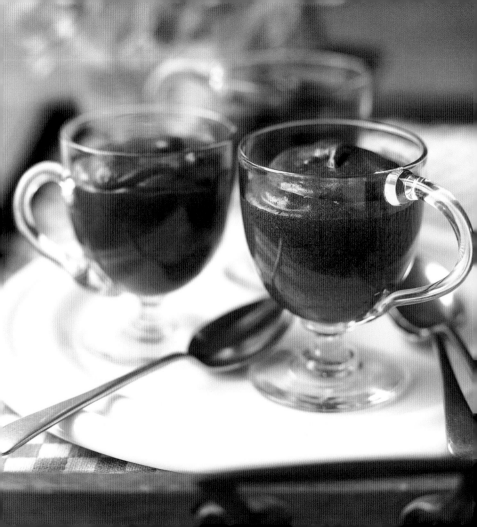

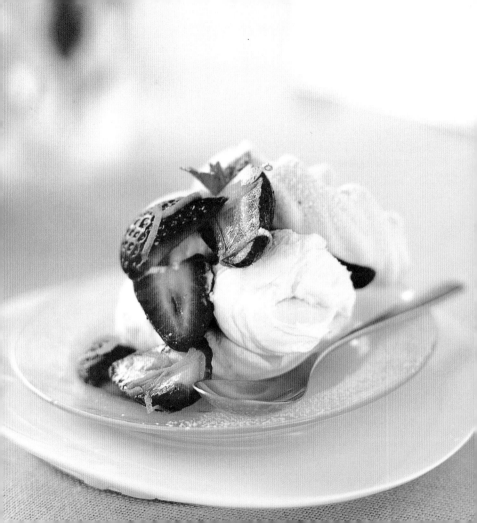

strawberries, meringue and mascarpone cream

250 g strawberries

freshly squeezed juice of
$^1/_2$ orange

2-3 tablespoons caster sugar

1 teaspoon grated unwaxed
orange zest

125 g mascarpone cheese

125 ml double cream

4 ready-made
meringue nests

fresh mint leaves, to serve

serves 2

Any shape of meringue can be used here, and chocolate meringues are good, too. This is also very pretty served in tall, thin glasses, with the meringue (perhaps broken into pieces), cream and fruit built up in layers.

Wash the strawberries and pat them dry, then hull, trim (cut in half if large) and put in a bowl. Squeeze over the orange juice. Add 1–1$^1/_2$ tablespoons sugar, to taste, and the orange zest. Stir gently until well blended, then set aside for at least 30 minutes or up to 6 hours.

Put the mascarpone in a bowl, then add the cream and 1–1$^1/_2$ tablespoons sugar, to taste. Whisk well, then cover and refrigerate until needed.

When ready to serve, put 1 meringue nest on each plate. Top with half the mascarpone cream mixture, then add half the strawberries. Put the remaining meringue nests on top, add the mint leaves and serve.

The best-quality chocolate, a hint of vanilla,
lots of frothy milk topped with whipped cream
and grated chocolate – this is the ultimate hot
drink for lovers.

the finest hot chocolate

*85 g plain chocolate,
broken into pieces*

*1 tablespoon caster sugar,
or to taste*

*1 vanilla pod, split
lengthways*

300 ml milk

*100 ml whipping cream,
whipped*

*freshly grated chocolate or
cocoa powder, for sprinkling*

2 mugs, warmed

serves 2

Put the chocolate pieces, sugar, vanilla pod and milk
in a small, heavy-based saucepan. Heat gently, stirring,
until the chocolate has melted, then bring to the boil,
whisking constantly with a balloon whisk, until very
smooth and frothy. Remove the vanilla pod.

Pour into warmed mugs, top with the whipped cream
and a sprinkling of freshly grated chocolate or cocoa
powder, and serve immediately.

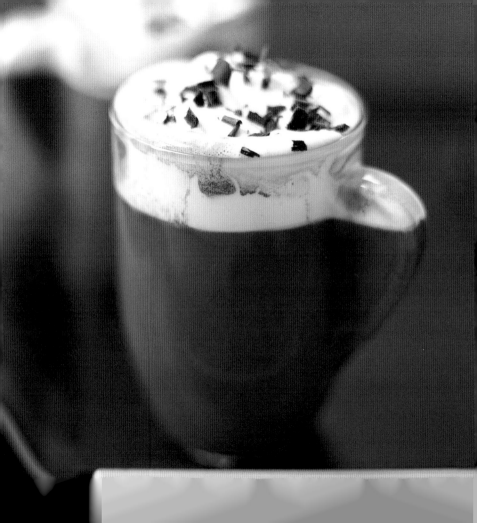

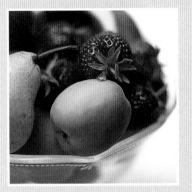

Little Treats

All mankind love a lover.
Ralph Waldo Emerson (1803–1882)

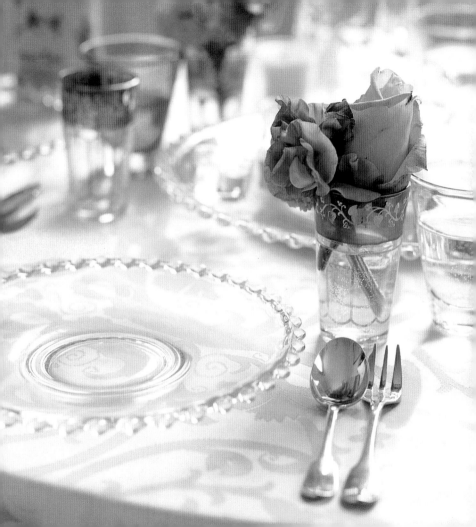

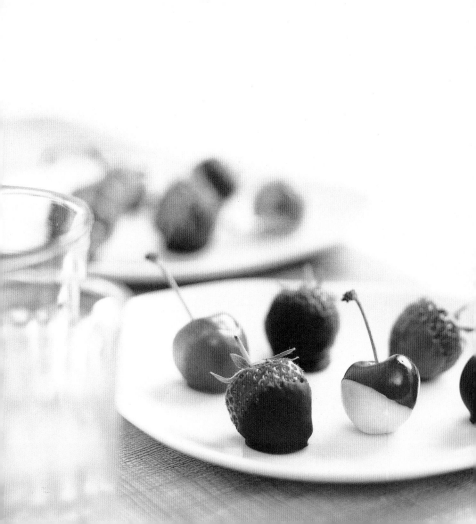

strawberries
and cherries *in chocolate*

250 g strawberries,
stalks on

250 g cherries, stalks on

30 g milk chocolate, broken
into small pieces

30 g white chocolate, broken
into small pieces

30 g plain chocolate, broken
into small pieces

greaseproof paper

mini paper muffin cases
(optional)

serves 4

Divide the strawberries and cherries into 3 equal piles.

Put the milk chocolate in a clean, dry heatproof bowl set over a saucepan of steaming but not boiling water and melt gently. Do not let the base of the bowl touch the water or let any water touch the chocolate, or the chocolate will 'seize' and be unusable.

Take one of the piles of fruit and dip them halfway into the melted chocolate, leaving the tops and stalks uncoated and visible. Transfer the fruit to greaseproof paper to set.

Melt the white and plain chocolate in the same way and dip 1 pile of each fruit into each type of chocolate. Chill the coated fruit for at least 1 hour.

To serve, peel off the greaseproof paper and put a selection of fruit in a mini muffin case. Alternatively, pile the fruit onto a large serving plate and help yourselves.

Make one of these and serve it with two spoons. Containing chocolate, banana, nuts and cherries, this sundae is sure to take your love life to new heights!

banana split

To make the chocolate sauce, heat the cream and sugar in a saucepan, then stir into the melted chocolate and mix well. Set aside.

To make the butterscotch sauce, put the sugar, cream and butter in a saucepan and stir over medium heat until melted and boiling. Reduce the heat and simmer for 3 minutes. Set aside.

Put the banana halves in the long, shallow glass dish. Put 3 scoops of ice cream along the length of the dish, between the 2 halves of banana. Drizzle 1 tablespoon each of the red berry sauce, chocolate sauce and butterscotch sauce over the top. Spoon the whipped cream around the base of the dish and over the ice cream. Sprinkle with chopped nuts and top with the cherries. If using wafers, set them in the ice cream at a jaunty angle.

1 ripe banana, halved lengthways

3 scoops of ice cream, one each of vanilla, chocolate and strawberry

1 tablespoon Red Berry Sauce (see page 20)

2–4 tablespoons whipped cream

1 tablespoon crushed mixed nuts

2–3 glacé cherries

2 wafers, to serve (optional)

chocolate sauce

250 ml double cream

4 tablespoons sugar

155 g bitter chocolate (70 per cent cocoa solids), melted (see page 51)

butterscotch sauce

100 g soft brown sugar

125 ml double cream

5 tablespoons butter

a long, shallow glass dish

makes 1, enough for 2 to share

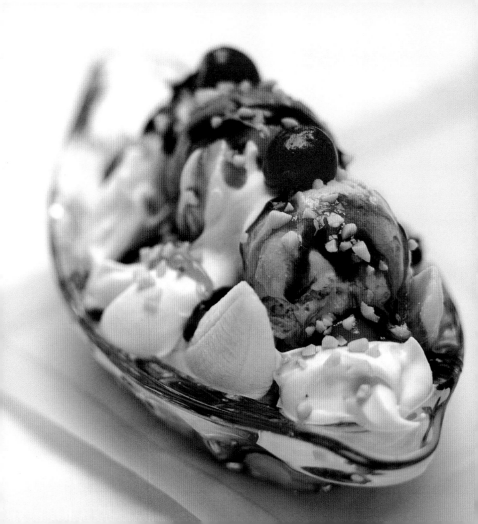

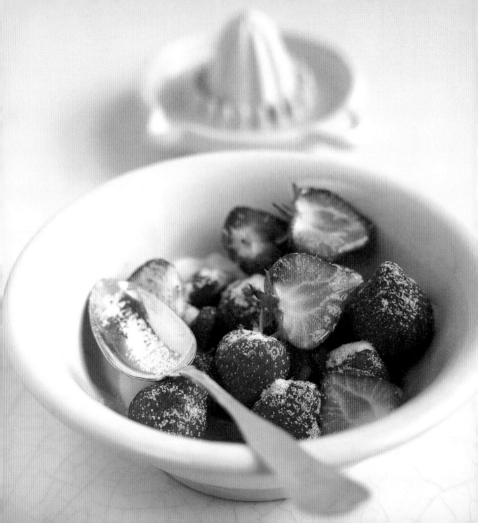

Succulent, juicy strawberries are the perfect summertime treat. Peach slices can be substituted for the strawberries, if you prefer.

sugared strawberries

1 kg strawberries, at room temperature

freshly squeezed juice of 1 lemon

3–5 tablespoons caster sugar

crème fraîche or whipped cream, to serve

serves 4–6

Trim the strawberries and put them in a pretty bowl. Add the lemon juice and 3 tablespoons sugar. Mix gently but thoroughly and let stand for about 15 minutes. Taste, and add more sugar if necessary.

This dish improves with standing, but don't leave it too long – about 1 hour is fine.

If using crème fraîche, sweeten it with 1 teaspoon caster sugar. Otherwise serve with whipped cream.

coffee and walnut kisses

These 'kisses' are delicate walnut and coffee biscuits sandwiched together with a rich chocolate-coffee ganache.

40 g walnut halves or pieces

100 g unsalted butter

70 g caster sugar

$^1/_2$ beaten egg

110 g self-raising flour, sifted

1 teaspoon instant coffee powder

ganache

100 g chocolate, broken into pieces

40 g unsalted butter

125 ml double cream

$1^1/_2$ teaspoons instant coffee powder

2 baking sheets covered with non-stick baking parchment

makes 24 biscuits, 12 'kisses'

Finely chop the walnuts – this is best done with a sharp knife to stop the nuts becoming oily.

Put the butter and sugar in a bowl and beat until creamy. Stir in the beaten egg and then fold in the sifted flour. Stir in the coffee powder, then the chopped walnuts. Put an even number of tablespoons of the mixture (about 24) onto the prepared baking sheets, spacing them well apart. Bake in a preheated oven at 180°C (350°F) Gas 4 for about 10 minutes, or until light brown around the edges. Remove from the oven, let cool and firm up on the tray for a couple of minutes, then carefully transfer to a wire rack and let cool completely.

Meanwhile, to make the ganache, put the chocolate, butter and cream in a saucepan and heat gently until the butter melts – do not let the mixture boil. Beat in the coffee powder. Remove the pan from the heat and stir with a wooden spoon. The mixture will thicken as it cools. Carefully sandwich the cool, fragile biscuits together with the ganache. Store in an airtight container for up to 3 days.

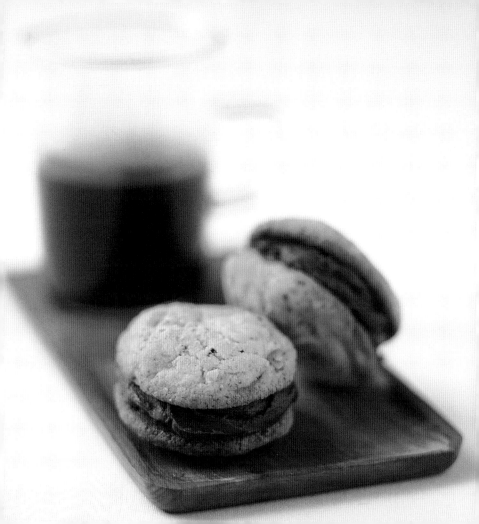

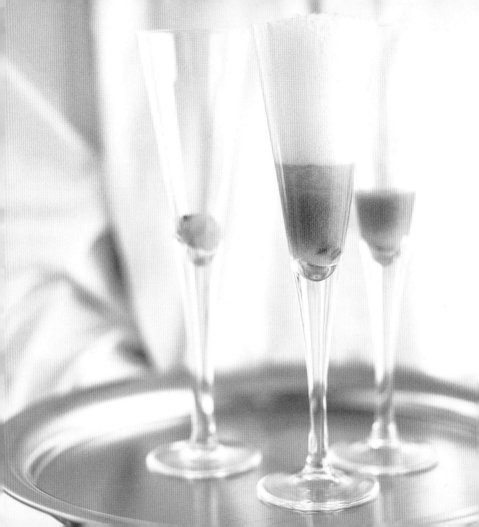

bellini

Peaches galore, topped up with champagne – this classic cocktail makes a wonderful tipple for lovers.

½ fresh peach, skinned

12.5 ml crème de pêche

a dash of peach bitters (optional)

champagne, to top up

peach ball, to garnish

makes 1

Put the peach in a blender and blend to a purée. Transfer the purée to a champagne flute. Pour in the crème de pêche and the peach bitters, if using, and gently top up with champagne, stirring carefully and continuously. Add a peach ball to the glass, then serve immediately.

This delicate cocktail combines ginger with champagne to delicious effect.

ginger champagne

2 thin slices of fresh root ginger

25 ml vodka

champagne, to top up

makes 1

Put the ginger in a shaker and press with a barspoon or muddler to release the flavour. Add some ice and the vodka, shake well and strain into a champagne flute. Top up with champagne and serve immediately.

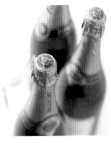

strawberry cosmopolitan

'Muddle' the ripe strawberries in a cocktail shaker using a barspoon, add the remaining ingredients and shake sharply. Strain into a frosted martini glass, garnish with ½ strawberry and serve.

3½ fresh strawberries, plus ½ to garnish

35 ml citrus vodka

25 ml Cointreau

15 ml freshly squeezed lime juice

a dash of cranberry juice (optional)

makes 1

cosmo royale

35 ml lemon vodka

15 ml freshly squeezed lime juice

15 ml Cointreau

50 ml cranberry juice

champagne, to float

orange zest, to garnish (optional)

makes 1

Put all the ingredients, except the champagne, in a cocktail shaker filled with ice. Shake sharply and strain into a frosted martini glass. Float the champagne on the surface and garnish with orange zest, if liked. Serve.

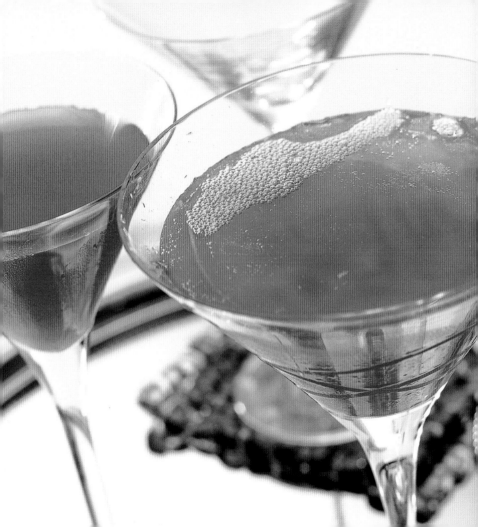

Index

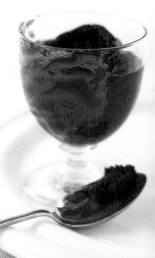

Credits

Key: *a=above, b=below, r=right, l=left, c=centre*

Recipes

Maxine Clark: *pages 25, 34, 41*
Linda Collister: *page 46*
Hattie Ellis: *page 56*
Clare Ferguson: *page 33*
Jane Noraika: *page 51*
Elsa Petersen-Schepelern: *pages 20, 52*
Louise Pickford: *pages 12, 15, 16, 18, 26*
Ben Reed: *pages 59, 60*
Sonia Stevenson: *page 29*
Laura Washburn: *pages 30, 38, 42, 45, 55*

Photographs

Martin Brigdale: *7al, 24, 28–35, 39–43, 47, 54, 63*
David Brittain: *36, 49, 64 background*
Peter Cassidy: *4–5, 10, 12*
Dan Duchars: *48*
Daniel Farmer: *11*
Tom Leighton: *endpapers*
William Lingwood: *50–51, 58–61*
David Loftus: *64c inset*
James Merrell: *7bl*
David Montgomery: *8l inset, 64l inset*
David Munns: *2–3, 44*
Noel Murphy: *64r inset*
Debi Treloar: *1, 20–23, 53, 57*
Ian Wallace: *13–18, 27*
Polly Wreford: *37*
Francesca Yorke: *6, 7ar & br, 8–9*

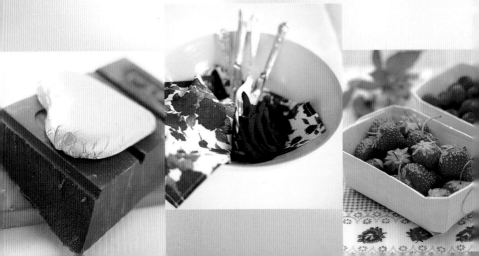

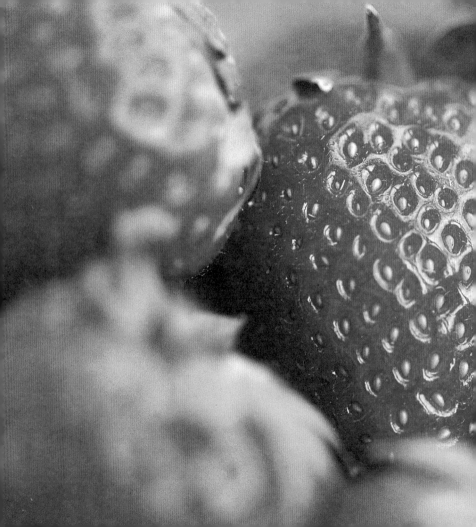